YOGA FOR BEGINNERS

The first step of Yoga practice. Essential requirements for health benefits. Improve your mind, body and spirit.

Elliot Wood

Copyright 2019 All rights reserved.

This document is geared towards providing exact and reliable information in regards to the topic and issue covered. The publication is sold with the idea that the publisher is not required to render accounting, officially permitted, or otherwise, qualified services. If advice is necessary, legal or professional, a practiced individual in the profession should be ordered.

- From a Declaration of Principles which was accepted and approved equally by a Committee of the American Bar Association and a Committee of Publishers and Associations.

In no way is it legal to reproduce, duplicate, or transmit any part of this document in either electronic means or in printed format. Recording of this publication is strictly prohibited and any storage of this document is not allowed unless with written permission from the publisher. All rights reserved.

The information provided herein is stated to be truthful and consistent, in that any liability, in terms of inattention or otherwise, by any usage or abuse of any policies, processes, or directions contained within is the solitary and utter responsibility of the recipient reader. Under no circumstances will any legal responsibility or blame be held against the publisher for any reparation, damages, or monetary loss due to the information herein, either directly or indirectly.

Respective authors own all copyrights not held by the publisher.

The information herein is offered for informational purposes solely, and is universal as so. The presentation of the information is without contract or any type of guarantee assurance.

The trademarks that are used are without any consent, and the publication of the trademark is without permission or backing by the trademark owner. All trademarks and brands within this book are for clarifying purposes only and are the owned by the owners themselves, not affiliated with this document.

Table of Contents

Chapter 1

Yoga For Beginners

Chapter 2

Common Myths About Yoga Practice

Chapter 3

Most Common Reasons Why You Must Start Yoga

Chapter 4

Health Benefits Of Yoga Practice

Chapter 5

What Clothes To Wear As A Yoga Beginners

Chapter 6

Yoga For Weight Loss

Chapter 7

Poses And Exercises In Yoga For Weight Loss

Chapter 8

How You Can Supercharge Your Diet With Easy Yoga Stretches

Chapter 9

Yoga For Stress Relief

Chapter 10

Yoga Poses For Stress Relief

Chapter 11

Yoga For Beginners To Ease Knee Pain

Chapter 12

How To Turn Yoga Into A Habit

Chapter 13

Yoga For Improving Your Mind, Body And Spirit

Chapter 14

Basic Yoga Routines For Beginners

Chapter 15

Considerations To Get The Most Out Of Your Yoga Practice

Chapter 16

Choosing Yoga Equipment As A Beginner

Chapter 17

Yoga For Overall Health And Weight Management

Chapter 18

Must Know Information For You As A Beginner

Chapter 19

Tips For Yoga Classes

INTRODUCTION

Yoga is the ancient form of exercise that is widely practiced today to stay fit and healthy. This form of art is not only popular for offering different physical benefits, but also known for improving mental, emotional and spiritual health.

Mastering in this form of exercise is certainly a step-by-step process. Yogis suggest that a beginner should always start practicing the easy postures first so that they can get the encouragement to continue further.

The basic postures are very easy to learn and practice which include sitting, standing and lying on different poses. But, it is very important to practice these easy postures with perfection to achieve the health benefits attached to it.

Medical practitioners and doctors also recommend their patients to practice the basic postures of this form of exercise regularly, owing to the exceptional therapeutic advantages attached to it.

Being a beginner, you will definitely notice several health benefits after practicing this art. Some of the basic and initial yoga for beginners are Kripalu and Viniyoga. Before you proceed with the advanced level it is very crucial to master these basic and simple postures first.

Being a beginner, you should always try to dedicate at least 15-20 minutes daily at the initial phase and gradually increase the timing of your practice which will increase the flexibility of joints, improve blood circulation and enhance lubrication.

Practicing the basic postures is must for all beginners as it prepares your body for the more difficult asanas. But, it is also equally important for practitioners to perform all the postures perfectly so that they can achieve all the health benefits easily.

Breathing exercises are the most important sessions for the beginners. Kapalbharti, Pranayama, and Anuloma-Viloma are few effective breathing exercises that a beginner should practice daily along with their regular workout session.

These exercises are mainly intended to improve the breathing patterns and also to improve the lung capacity. With these breathing exercises you will surely feel rejuvenated and relaxed. Being the great stress busters, these breathing exercises help you to get rid of anxiety, worries and daily tensions.

Moreover, a beginner should know the yoga etiquettes before start practicing this form of art. You may seek help from some expert professionals or Yogis who will not only teach you the basic postures of this exercise, but also teach you the basic etiquettes of this form of art.

Being a beginner, it is always recommended to start with basic and simple stretches like back bends, finishing poses, twist, supine, balance poses, standing and sitting postures.

Practicing this form of art in the early morning is always recommended and before practicing it is always better to take a bath. Yogis also suggest that practitioners should end up their workout sessions with Shavasana.

It is advisable that practitioners should not eat food at least one hour prior to their practice. Wearing loose and comfortable gears is also necessary for a workout session so that you feel comfortable and easy while practicing the poster.

This BEGINNERS GUIDE will enlighten you with some of the crucial aspects that a beginner should keep in mind before they start practicing their yoga postures.

Happy Reading.

CHAPTER 1

Yoga For Beginners

Yoga can be a fun and exciting way to get your body in shape and your muscles stronger than they have ever been. Yoga uses the body's own weight to help increase muscle strength while stretching the muscles to give them a lean appearance.

Yoga is often erroneously viewed as a less strenuous activity than other exercises that are typically done in a gym. Many people make the mistake of thinking that they are not pushing their bodies as hard as they truly are during a yoga class.

Yoga teaches us how to maintain harmony between various forces acting on our body. In case, we are not taking care of our body, yoga shows us the way to restore our health by taking control of our mind and body. It is in our hands to take charge of our body. There are certain yoga basics which should be followed while practicing yoga.

Beginners should not make very ambitious plans as yoga requires patience. Set realistic targets and achieve them, it provides motivation for continuing yoga practice. For beginners, 30 minutes to one hour of yoga practice is adequate. Do not expect miracles overnight. Do not strain yourself while doing asanas.

Your progress in yoga will depend on your age and health at the time of starting yoga. One month of yoga practice can show positive results for most of the beginners. Practice yoga in a neat and well ventilated room by putting a yoga mat on the floor. If weather is comfortable, practicing yoga in a lawn early in the morning can be a wonderful experience.

It is recommended to have a fixed time each day for yoga practice. One to two hours before sunrise is the ideal time for yoga practice as oxygen content is high and there are no distractions. As per your convenience, yoga can be practiced in evening also provided you are not too much tired. Do not eat anything three hours before doing yoga.

Yoga is not designed to make the muscles ache or the body to feel intense pain that often comes with weight training or cardiovascular exercise. Individuals who takes a beginner yoga class for the first time will more than likely feel a burn in their muscles a few hours after they have finished the class.

A person may want to keep a journal about his or her yoga experience. These journals may detail the exercises that were performed each day and the ways in which the exercises affected the participant's body the next day and the days afterward. This is a great way for someone to be able to look back and see how far he or she has come with strengthening his or her body through yoga.

Once someone has taken the beginner yoga class for a few months, he or she should find it much easier to do. At this time, a person may want to try a more difficult class or take the same class more frequently. As the body strengthens, it will need to be pushed harder and in new ways in order to progress and become stronger.

Constipation is one of the ailments which can prevent you from enjoying full benefits of yoga. Drink enough water and include sufficient fiber in your food to avoid constipation. Your bowels should be clear in the morning before yoga practice.

Yoga practice is not complete if mind keeps wandering. For most of the asanas concentrate on the body part being affected by that asana or on your breathing. A peaceful mind is essential for gaining perfect health, strength and vitality.

Essentially yoga practice involves the following aspects:

- Restraining of senses.
- Following a simple diet.
- Controlling the mind.
- Proper breathing and relaxation.
- Regular exercise.
- Regular meditation.
- Continuous introspection to identify your weaknesses for self-improvement.

CHAPTER 2

Common Myths About Yoga Practice

Yoga is a very popular form of exercising and spiritual balancing, but it is also very often understood by a lot of people. This is almost inevitable when you consider the incredible popularity of Yoga as a discipline and the many different strands that Yoga has.

Quite often people have experience with one type of Yoga but not another, and as such they will base their overall impression of Yoga on what they have seen.

It is like people basing their impression on Germans on the most famous German they know - Adolf Hitler, or more recently the portrayal of George Bush internationally as the only example of an American anyone knows.

The truth is that Yoga can be very different depending on who you learn it from and how they perceive Yoga. This chapter looks at learning yoga for beginners and some of the common misconceptions therein.

One: Yoga is a form of exercise.

Well yes it is, but so is walking. I can walk from my couch to my table and I can hardly claim to have done my exercise for the day. The truth is that exercise is just the beginning of what yoga is.

It's closer to a combination of exercise, physiotherapy, psychology and spirituality all rolled into one. As you come to master Yoga you will need to become more and more mentally strong, and most importantly disciplined.

If you can discipline yourself to do regular Yoga sessions, and maintain your discipline to do each pose for the prescribed time, and do it properly, then you will naturally become a very disciplined and organized person.

For some people this transcends to a spiritual level because they are so efficient and clearing their thoughts while meditating.

Two: Yoga is for Hippies.

As previously mentioned Yoga can be a very spiritual experience if you become good enough at clearing your thoughts and concentrating whilst performing the exercises. But you certainly do not have to begin with any spiritual belief. Yoga believes in aligning the body and the mind and the spirit through achieving inner balance.

What that means to you is probably going to depend entirely on what your beliefs already are. For some people it will be a spiritually freeing experience, for others it will be an effective way of distressing and achieving a level of calmness of thought. Still others will claim that these things are one and the same.

Three: Yoga is a fad.

Recently there have been some very hyped up Yoga courses making big claims about what Yoga can achieve. These are easy to associate with other 'fad' exercise crazes. However Yoga is not something new and is based in documents that are hundreds

Four: Yoga is too slow to help me lose weight/gain tone etc.

This one is way off the mark, but we have been somewhat trained by the weight loss industry that weight loss, and toning our body is all about hours in the gym and fast high impact exercise. That's simply not true. Yoga can help with weight loss and in particularly toning for a number of reasons.

Firstly the exercises, while low impact and performed either statically or slowly - are still exercises. While you use them you are using your muscles, and in many cases you are using muscles and muscle groups that regular exercise programs ignore.

The second way that Yoga can be of benefit in a weight loss program is that it will increase your mental strength and allow you to be more disciplined with your food consumption. When it comes down to it excess weight is a result of excess eating and not enough physical exercise to burn off those calories.

Have you ever noticed how some people can eat donut after donut and not put on any weight at all? It seems unfair, but it's a natural result of the state of their body. Usually these people will be quite 'sinewy' and this muscle allows them the metabolize food faster.

That's the third benefit of Yoga in weight loss, as your muscles develop your body will actually become more efficient at consuming foods and processing them into nutrients and waste.

CHAPTER 3

Most Common Reasons Why You Must Start Yoga

There are many reasons why you may think about starting yoga. Here are seven common reasons why you may want to start to learn yoga. Maybe one of these reasons applies to you.

1. Yoga for Stress Relief.

A gentle yoga practice at the end of a stressful day is the ideal way to unwind and relieve tension from your body. This has to be the most popular reason why you start yoga. Your life is busy and full of conflicting demands.

The constant hustle and bustle of modern day life means you have trouble switching off and relaxing. The essence of yoga is to encourage you to relax, take time out of your busy schedule and be present and focus on your breath. This instantly calms your mind and relaxes your body.

2. Yoga for Back Pain Relief

Have you ever suffered back pain or experienced sore, tense muscles? Yoga exercises are designed to gently stretch your muscles, increase the range of flexibility in your joints and bring suppleness to your spine. For example, yoga poses, such as the cobra, the locust or seated forward bend, all help to soothe your aching back.

3. Yoga for Inner Peace and Calm

If you are going through an emotional crisis or recovering from a severe illness, chances are you feel unhappy and unsettled about your situation.

When you feel unhappy or down, your mind is agitated and it takes longer for the body to heal. Yoga breathing exercises and meditation practices help to promote a sense of ease and calm within the body and mind.

4. Yoga for Weight Loss

Yoga is the ideal exercise to encourage you to lose weight and develop positive eating habits. Yoga philosophy promotes a vegetarian diet based on natural, unprocessed foods.

In addition, yoga encourages you to be conscious of how you eat. Prior to eating, you bless your food and Give Thanks to the hands and souls who worked to grow your food and deliver it to your local supermarket.

This sense of reverence and respect for what you eat and how you eat means you take time to select foods which nurture and nourish your body. Instead of mindlessly eating foods, on-the-go, or in front of the TV, from a yogic perspective, you consciously chew each morsel, the more you chew and take time to enjoy and digest your food, and the deeper is your sense of fulfillment from eating.

5. Yoga for Personal Development

Underpinning the physical aspects of yoga is a philosophy and way of living your life which guides you towards enlightenment. The ultimate goal of yoga is to unite with the divine and live a life of harmony and inner calm.

The Yoga Sutras offers you a broad range of ethical and practical guidelines to living a healthy harmonious life. Many students gain inner strength, clarity and awareness of themselves through studying The Yoga Sutras

6. Yoga for Energy

Have you ever felt tired and zapped of energy? Yoga exercises can be used to stimulate and energise your mind and body. Blocked energy is released through the chakras, which correspond to key nerve centres or plexuses in the body. As the blocked energy is released you feel energised and revitalised.

7. Yoga for Health

Yoga offers you a truly holistic way of living your life. The physical postures promote a strong and healthy body, the philosophical guidelines offer you a simple natural way to experience life, meditation practices and breathing exercises all promote vitality and ease and comfort within your body.

As you can see, there are many reasons why you may consider practicing yoga. All reasons are valid. If you are thinking of starting yoga, take your time to find a qualified yoga teacher and enjoy your yoga journey. of years old which describe exercises and poses that were probably being performed for generations before that.

An individual style of Yoga may come and go, but as long as people are still stretching before a game of football then Yoga will still be being used.

CHAPTER 4

Health Benefits Of Yoga Practice

Most people who actually benefit from Yoga are those who practice, and continue to practice. Often times beginners try Yoga once and never again. They do not see how doing stretches or putting their body in uncomfortable poses helps their life. Here are 5 reasons why us Yoga lovers love the practice:

1. Yoga Relaxes:

When you practice yoga, your full attention is required. The practice allows you to detach from your long, hard day and turn in. For an hour or so, your practice requires you to be in the present moment.

Most of the day, we are busy working, or making plans, or thinking about where we need to go, what we need to do... During this hour or so, your mind must focus and detach from all those things that you did or have to do because in order to do any pose, or listen to the instructor's direction, you need to pay attention.

By leaving your work load behind or skipping through your thoughts about your "must do's," for that hour, you are clearing your mind. When your mind is clear, you can better reflect on the past, plan your future, and enjoy your present moment.

2. Yoga Strengthens the Body:

Yoga is workout - Of The Mind. There is no doubt that Yoga postures and poses strengthen your muscles and help you lose weight and manage cellulite. It also depends on how often you practice (on and off your mat). Practicing on a regular basis will strengthen those more than others.

Yoga allows you to learn about your own body. Which poses can you do? Which poses do you like or dislike? It teaches you your physical limitations, physical capabilities, and physical preferences. How can you strengthen your body without first learning about your very own first?

By practicing, you are able to find out if you are a back-bender, arm balancer, or both. I can tell you, I never considered myself flexible before I began to practice Yoga.

Over time, I discovered that I am much more flexible than I thought (in my body and my mind). Being flexible and open in the mind, allows you to be flexible and open in your body. Try it, you have everything to gain.

3. Yoga Strengthens the Mind:

Simple- "Healthy Body = Healthy Mind." Yoga offers us the tools that help us think clearly. You say, "How can going upside down help me clear my mind?" Well, actually, going upside down reverses your blood flow to your brain which washes out the old and pumps the new and fresh.

Besides that, the practice of Yoga (asana) has everything to take with you off your mat. For example, as you practice, one goal is to keep your body engaged, yet soft. We call this Sthira-Sukha. (Sthira - Firm and Alert) and (Sukha- Ease and without Tension). Sound like a piece of cake? Think again.

Our practice helps us to find this balance because by finding this balance, we can advance our practice. Otherwise, poses simply remain poses. Think about how this could benefit life outside your mat.

In your workplace, employers favor those who have the ability to lead, be strong and firm, speak up, be quick (qualities that Sthira brings) BUT- they also need those who remain calm during crisis, have problem-solving abilities, are polite, communicate well with others (qualities that Sukha brings). Wouldn't having both benefit you in your work place? Absolutely.

4. Yoga Teaches you to Prevent:

Not only does Yoga help you reflect and sort out all of your issues (even the ones you did not realize you had), but it also helps you to prevent future problems in your life. Yoga enhances your thinking skills. Sometimes, we like to do things over and over again and hope or expect a different result each time (definition of insanity).

I know that I am guilty of it as well. Yoga practice is that little light bulb that pops in your head and tells you, "hey, maybe I should try something different since this clearly is not working." So, you may ask, "how can doing a yoga pose possibly help me with this.?"

Here is why: Since the poses teach you about your body, they also teach you how far you can go or if perhaps you have gone too far. If your body does not feel good in a pose or causes you pain, you are asked to COME OUT and try a different or modified pose that is better for your body. See the connection? A lot of times these concepts are not even noticed.

We begin to say, "Yoga feels good, puts me in a better mood, changed my life.. etc" It is because as we begin to practice, we begin to recognize the things that are getting in our way and we recognize them more quickly than before, then by having a clear mind, we take action. Over time, this becomes a prevention tool.

5. Yoga Changes Old Habits:

You know those bad habits you have and find a very hard time stepping away from them? Well, here is where Yoga can help you in that area of your life. Yoga practice makes you recognize all sorts of things about yourself that you did not know.

Simply because, as mentioned before, it requires your full attention. Once you learn about yourself, you recognize your habits (the good and bad ones).

As you may know, the first step in changing anything is recognizing the problem. In this case, recognizing your bad habits. Sometimes we are not fully aware of our habits. So how can we change them if we do not even know we have them?

By practicing Yoga, we learn about our body, preferences, and our health. Naturally, paying close attention to ourselves is like studying our own self and seeing ourself through the eyes of the world outside of us. This is not so easy to do, especially if we are so caught up in our stressful and busy lives.

As we practice over time, we become extremely sensitive to notice everything about ourselves and that is when we clearly recognize our habits. To go into more depth, we begin to recognize how we could possibly make our habits better or shift things in other areas to help balance out the things that we cannot change.

For example, excessive smokers or drinkers who wish they could stop their habits may find it almost impossible to let go. Working with your body, over time teaches the concept of "letting go of that which does not serve me." Over time, with practice and most importantly commitment, change will come and it will come naturally.

CHAPTER 5

What Clothes To Wear As A Yoga Beginner

So, after hearing of the endless health benefits from Yoga and the assurances that nobody expects you to sit with your ankle behind you head on the first lessons, you have signed up to a Yoga for beginners lesson and are ready to go.

And then it hits you: What clothes should you wear to a Yoga class? What equipment do you need? And most importantly, how do you get hold of it on time for your lesson? Relax: You probably already own everything you need, or can get it with a quick visit to your nearest sports store.

Clothes

When buying yoga clothes the key word is comfort. You need to be able to comfortably move and bend without the clothes being so tight they stop you, but they need to be tight enough so you don't trip on them. In some cases you can use loose gym pants for your Yoga lessons with no problems.

Depending on the type of Yoga lessons you are attending you may want to buy something that is easy to wash; for example, if you are practicing Bikram Yoga you will be in a heated room, and sweat a lot, so synthetic fibres may soon become uncomfortable. Loose cotton pants and a t-shirt that is long enough for you to bend without being afraid of showing off too much flesh is often more than enough equipment for your Yoga class.

You can choose to wear shorts or long pants, depending on what makes you more comfortable. Most people choose light or neutral coloured clothes, as wearing bright colours may be distracting, but there are no hard set rules about that.

Shoes

Most people practice Yoga barefoot, but if you are attending a yoga studio is worth getting a pair of gym slippers for comfort while walking around to get to the room where your lesson is taking place. If you are uncomfortable barefoot you can use Yoga socks to cover your feet as well.

Towels and Accessories

Some people choose to wear accessories that help them connect better with the spiritual aspects of Yoga, such as bracelets or pendants with a special meaning, but this is completely optional.

If you are a beginner you may want to bring some towels that you can fold to help support your body when practicing some forms, but if you are attending a Yoga for beginners class your teacher will most probably already taken that into account.

CHAPTER 6

Yoga For Weight Loss

There are a lot of ways that you can lose your extra pounds and you might have already heard of yoga for weight loss. However, you are a little worried whether this is something that you should try because you are really not that familiar with the techniques.

You also think that you are not flexible enough so that you can execute the routines. And because of these, you thought that this is something that can only be done by certain people.

When trying yoga for weight loss, you will realize that this is actually one of the most effective ways that you can have a better figure. This is because it can help you increase your body's flexibility and to reduce fat. A lot of experts believe that this is very effective especially since a lot of people have already benefited through it.

This is also very convenient because you can do it right in the comforts of your home. You will no longer need to go to the gym or use very heavy equipment. As a matter of fact, the only thing that you need is a small space and a mat where you can lay and sit. This also does not require a huge chunk of your time because you can do a simple routine in just about 30 minutes every day.

But if you are going to try it out, you need to know that there are also some things that you still need to take into account. For instance, yoga for weight loss can be done on your own.

However, if this is your first time, it is much better if you are as-

sisted by a coach
or a trainer. This way, you will be taught about the proper forms and executions of the routines. Anyway, as soon as you have learned the basics, you can continue to do it on your own.

In general, there is a need for you to be familiar with the routines. This is because it involves a large number of intensive but low-impact exercises.

Usually, it is characterized by stretching and conditioning that requires great flexibility from you. This can actually be very helpful in promoting better blood circulation which can be very helpful for a better digestion.

However, you should also know that the results that you can get from this kind of exercise are not as drastic as you might have expected. In general, you can only burn about 150 to 300 calories in an hour-long routine. Nevertheless, you are assured that this can be a steady approach so that you can lose your excess fats slowly.

You also need to know that you cannot just depend on yoga for weight loss. It is still necessary that you have a very healthy meal plan. You have to make sure that you are burning more calories than what you are taking in.

When trying yoga for weight loss, it is also a good idea if you become a part of a group so that you can keep motivating each other towards your goal of achieving a slimmer figure.

We mentioned earlier that yoga is a form of physical and mental discipline, so doing yoga will provide you with the best results in this regard. There are various types of yoga and Iyengar yoga is one of the very popular yoga that helps in building muscles and thus, improves your body posture.

However, while going to practice yoga, always make sure that you practice this form of physical exercise under the supervision of yoga experts to get better results.

In order to lose excessive weight, vinyasa or flow yoga is recommended which is based on the performance of a series of yoga poses known as sun salutations. It incorporates various popular, athletic and sweat-drenched styles of yoga. Practicing ashtanga, power yoga and hot yoga also provide great weight loss results.

The ashtanga yoga is dynamic style of yoga with certain advantages for the people who are looking for some useful ways to lose their excessive weight. The practitioners of this particular style of yoga are considered to be the most dedicated yogis.

The best thing about this style of yoga is that one can easily practice it at their home. When it comes to power yoga which is very famous among people provides strong cardiovascular workout to its practitioners. While the vinyasa yoga is done in a hot room to ensure that you will sweat during its practice. So, yoga for weight loss is the best way.

At the end we can say that practicing yoga is not only recommended to those who are overweight, but also to all to have a healthy and prosperous life.

Reasons You Should Use Yoga For Weight Loss

Yoga for weight loss is not a common topic on the minds of people who regularly partake in yoga. People start practicing Yoga because it is one of the easiest ways to live a stress free lifestyle. Yoga helps protect you from the grime of everyday life and releases all of the pressure and stress you might be feeling. However, there are 3 very good reasons why you should start practicing Yoga if you want to lose weight.

1. Enjoy an improvement of overall health

When you start practicing Yoga for weight loss, you will not only be losing weight but also improving your overall health. Yoga helps you to condition your internal systems and organs, in addition to helping you get rid of any extra fat your body might be storing. Yoga isn't a short term solution.

You will notice that once you start losing weight, your body will improve, your health will improve and you will become much fitter. Yoga is so much more than just a body improvement, it also helps you become spiritually and mentally more healthy.

There are no negative side effects.

Your body is pre-programmed with a blue print of what perfect health is. Your body is constantly struggling to get back to this state of perfect health. It is up to us - as masters of our bodies - to return our body into that perfect shape.

Yoga was designed in mind to make sure that we can easily return to the perfect state of health that our body craves.

Yoga is about working holistically with your body. You won't be just fixing one problem, you'll be fixing many. You will also find that you will have less exercise injuries when practicing Yoga for weight loss. A lot of exercising forms will actually injure your body because of pushing your muscles in an unnatural way.

Achieve permanent weight loss with Yoga.

There have been a lot of studies that have been performed over the years, and it has been shown that those people who have lost weight by practicing Yoga actually lose weight permanently. If you use chemicals or other gimmicks that are often being sold to the public, you will eventually pick up this weight again because you lost it unnaturally.

With Yoga, if you maintain a healthy diet and practice Yoga for weight loss, you will keep the weight off for the rest of your life. Yoga helps you to tackle the mental and physical problems for your weight gain. If you are obese or overweight, there is normally a problem you are struggling with. Yoga helps you identify these problems and work through them.

CHAPTER 7

Poses And Exercises In Yoga For Weight Loss

Practicing yoga not only helps in toning your body, improving the physical and mental wellbeing, but also helps in fat loss. Yoga for weight loss is very commonly used by most of the people as the awareness is spreading. Many celebrities are using yoga for weight loss nowadays.

Yoga is an effective way to maintain healthy body without any negative side effects. It helps in reducing the fat and increasing the metabolism of the body. There are various school and styles of yoga which depict different ways of practicing yoga.

Some of the styles are: Bikram, Kundalini, Astanga and Iyengar. They all aim towards the same goal but in slightly different ways. There are many poses or asanas in yoga for weight loss. Deep breathing in yoga increases the intake of oxygen in the body. Some of the poses and exercises in yoga for weight loss are as below:

1. Pranayam: Pranayam is a set of breathing exercises that have an effective impact on weight loss. Deep breathing done in the proper way helps in reducing the abdominal fat. There are different breathing techniques which can be practiced like kapalbhati, bhastrika, anulom vilom, bharamari and ujjayi pranayam.

Kapalbhati is said to be very effective since it involves forceful exhalation of air. Care should be taken that this should be done on an empty stomach only. This is not only good for obesity but also for indigestion and acidity.

In Anulom Vilom, one has to close one nostril with the thumb and breathe deeply from the other. This has to be repeated alternating the nostrils. These deep breathing exercises are very helpful and should be done under guidance.

2. Sun Salutations: Sun Salutations or Surya Namaskar is a series of 12 poses which help in weight loss and tone up the whole body. These poses along with sequenced breathing provide a lot of benefits to the body and mind. One should start with 1 or 2 rounds and slowly increase to at least 10 to 12 rounds. People with high blood pressure and pregnant women are advised not to perform this.

Saluting the sun: This can also be called "surya namaskar"; and this is how it is done;

1. Stand with your feet joined together and part of your soles in the ground; at the same time, fold your hands in front of your chest.

Raise your palms above your head and bend backwards; then, breathe out and at the same time, bend your waist with your hands at your sides and your palms to the ground. I advise you not to bend your knees, but touch them with your forehead. After sometime, you rise slowly with your back straight and your finger tips to the ground.

2. Still in that position, stretch your left foot to the back using your fingertips as its support; then, position your right foot as you did the left with your feet flat on the ground. Let your head be bent and hanging.

Take a slanting plank position with your weight on your arms and your toes; let your chest, knees and chin touch the ground with your back yard (butt) in the air. The next step is to take a semi-plank solution and repeat the former positions.

You can repeat for as long as you wish.

There are other forms of yoga for weight loss such as crescent pose, ashtanga pose, and the bikram pose. These poses are very good for weight loss, and note that when they are combined with other exercises like cardio exercise, they will yield tremendous results, and you will have cause to smile.

3. Bhujanga Asana: This is also called the Cobra Pose. It works on the shoulders, back, arms and other internal organs.

4. Yoga Spinal Twists: This works on your abdominal region and your entire digestive system. Spinal Twists help in burning calories and toning the abs. This is a good yoga for weight loss. Likewise there are many other poses which help in weight loss. One has to learn under guidance and perform slowly.

Yoga for weight loss will be effective only if combined with a proper diet. Eliminate the junk food and carbonated drinks from your diet. Include lot of greens, pulses, sprout, salads and fruits in your food intake to provide the body with the necessary proteins and vitamins. Do not break your yoga routine; do it regularly with dedication.

The results may not be very quick but be patient and keep practicing yoga for weight loss. It is important to do yoga under an expert's guidance. Yoga for weight loss will also result in a toned body, flexible body, less stress and anxiety, increase in concentration, strengthening of physical and mental health.

CHAPTER 8

How You Can Supercharge Your Diet With Easy Yoga Stretches

Studies reveal that yoga not only helps in losing weight, when coupled with a well-chosen diet, of course, but also reduces stress levels. By reducing the hormones released during stress, our body is signaled to increase insulin which in turn tells our body to burn what we've eaten instead of storing it as fat.

How and why does yoga assist in losing weight?

It provides cardiovascular workout which in fact is exercise-but in a relaxing manner. It doesn't burn calories as rapid as the fast-paced, rigid workouts, but it does its work slowly and surely as long as you regularly follow the routine. Two of the most popular yoga types recommended for weight loss is the Bikram Yoga and the Ashtanga Yoga.

These forms combine the meditative yoga breathing techniques with fast, active movements. Bikram Yoga mixes calmer yoga postures with cardiovascular and aerobic workout. It also uses heat as an integral part of the exercises in helping you to sweat out the toxins.

The speed of the cardio takes a while to get used to. Nevertheless, it helps quickly deal with losing weight. Ashtanga Yoga or eight-limb exercise, on the other hand, uses a series of complicated yoga postures harmonized with breathing. This is more for those in the advanced level already. It produces internal heat that leads you to sweat out profusely, thereby detoxifying your body.

Essentially, the yoga postures encourage metabolism, calorie burning, respiratory balance, and as mentioned earlier, lowers stress. Not only does it help you lose weight, it keeps the weight off through continued practice.

It also strengthens your muscles, tones your body, and, best of all, it forges a powerful connection between your mind and body. Yoga weight loss does not happen almost immediately though, you have to spend long hours following the routine to succeed.

Determination, patience, and self-control is a must for those who wish want to try yoga. But before you do try, as a beginner, you must consult a yoga instructor or your health care provider first to help you determine which type of yoga will suit you best.

From there, you can work up to the level that you would like to proceed with. All forms of yoga share one common goal: to balance your mind and body - increasing your self-awareness and providing you with a sense of calmness which will eventually guide you to practice restraint over cravings, anxiety, even depression, the usual causes of weight gain.

Yoga is not a calling for everyone, but if you think it's yours, then go ahead and start now. If nothing else, you'll enjoy the certain relaxation.

While the exercises and actual poses compared to traditional aerobic exercises will not burn as many calories, yoga weight loss has been shown in medical research to occur when combined with other exercise programs and proper diets. Unwanted flab will disappear as yoga promotes toning of the muscles, increased flexibility and improved blood circulation.

The desire to change your lifestyle comes through yoga which in turn leads to weight loss. Your destructive eating patterns and habits will ultimately change as your thought process regarding food changes.

With the strong connection of body-mind, you will become more in tune with what you eat and how you feel once you are finished.

Yoga weight loss happens as your mind becomes focused enough to let you examine the bad eating habits that led you to eat the unhealthy food that causes weight gain and leaves your body feeling sluggish.

Physical activity along with the focus of the mind plays a very important role in weight loss. Your body is completely detoxified through yoga by stretching and massaging organs, joints and muscles. Your system can flush out harmful toxins in your body that are voided through this body detoxification process.

You will experience a new found energy for life, after flushing out the system and will be more up to staying fit and exercising on a regular basis. Extreme yoga, which is an Americanized version of yoga, can be practiced once you get used to the poses; also known as power yoga, it offers the potential of extreme fat-burning.

Preventing weight gain is obvious through yoga, however when practiced properly and frequently it can also promote weight loss. Gaining peace and happiness in your life comes from yoga, and it's a fantastic introduction into the world of fitness

CHAPTER 9

Yoga For Stress Relief

Yoga breathing is called pranayama. Pranayama (or "control of the life force"), also literally translated as, "breath control," is just that. Controlled breathing in different styles has a detectable, and welcomed effect, on the psyche and the body.

Slow the heart rate, feel less out of breath, and relax your muscles, beginning with your breath. Research has shown that yoga breathing techniques are beneficial treatment for stress and stress-related problems. The mind is calmed, and the judgment is clearer, as yoga breathing is practiced on a regular basis.

Yoga breathing involves a range of deep, slow, rhythmic breaths. If you pay attention to your breath, when you are stressed, it will be irregular, shallow, nervous, and jagged. This happens involuntarily as a response to stress, but this rapid, shallow breathing actually amplifies stress levels.

The result is a vicious cycle that can climax into a panic attack for those with anxiety disorders. Practice controlled breathing, daily, as a stress management technique. This breathing can be done anywhere, at any time.

Breath control, combined with Hatha yoga poses, stretches and strengthens the muscles of the body. Stress often triggers muscle clenching, spasms, and an overall aching discomfort in the body. Poses, such as the mountain pose, supported bridge pose, child's pose, and happy baby pose, are all excellent for relaxation and stress relief.

Depending upon the lesson plan, each session of Hatha yoga can involve from 10 to 70 poses. Yoga instructors often end each class with Sivasana (Corpse Pose). This pose finishes up many classes because of the relaxing properties.

Through regular yoga practice, the body is also better supported, throughout the day, in posture, strength, and flexibility. Yoga relieves fatigue and helps you feel more energized. When a person feels physically stronger and more able, the emotional benefits are extraordinary. It's much easier to go out and face the day and put stress on the "back burner."

The Benefits Of Yoga For Stress Relief

The benefits of physical activity for mental, emotional, and physical health have been praised over the years, and Yoga is the oldest existing structured method for relieving stress. Some businesses have even started implementing corporate Yoga fitness programs to improve overall employee wellbeing.

When you consider reduced stress, increased morale, better employee attendance, and the perceived benefit among employees, a corporate Yoga program is not expensive; and some employees are willing to co-pay for these classes.

While the stereotype in most business decision makers' minds might be the room full of Yoga participants moving and breathing as one, these routines are deeply personalized, and exercises can be tailored for any individual looking to relieve stress.

Controlled breathing is one of the key aspects of any Yoga posture. Erratic breathing patterns frequently accompany stressful physical responses, so learning to master this physical response can alleviate some of the stress in a tense situation. For individuals experiencing chronic anxiety, gaining control of breathing can be an important step in gaining control of other factors.

Yoga promotes self-awareness at the level of the individual muscles. Many individuals are unaware of the full extent of muscle tension within their bodies. Unfortunately, runaway muscle tension can lead to persistent aches, pain, and emotional agitation. Muscle tension is just pent up energy screaming to be used.

Hatha, and other physical forms Yoga, were designed to release energy, constructively. Yogic awareness, stretching, relaxing, and strengthening of the muscles will allow the individual to first notice the problem area, while exercising mental, physical, and emotional control with accuracy.

It has been noted that those, who regularly participate in a structured Yoga session, have lower cortisol levels. Cortisol is one of the body's responses to stress, and it has been recorded that individuals reporting less stress have lower cortisol levels.

Increased self-confidence has often been linked with lower stress levels, and many aspects of Yoga have been linked to increased self-confidence. Regular Yoga participants noted increased muscle strength, increased flexibility, improved stamina, and improved balance. These physical measures of self-development can promote stress relief.

Most photographs promote the idea of holding poses for long periods of time. This is true for styles, such as Restorative and Iyengar Yoga. Yet, there are also forms of Yoga that leave many participants drenched in sweat. It is no secret that physical exercise relieves stress, and some forms of Vinyasa, Flow, Power, and Hot Yoga can be very intense physical workouts.

Doing yoga for stress relief doesn't have to be an involved routine. If you don't have time to do a full yoga routine, use the separate parts of yoga to relax and rejuvenate.

Deep breathing, meditation and poses can go a long way toward conquering stress. Simple yoga techniques take minutes to do and can be incorporated into your exercise routine. You can also do them whenever stress takes its toll to regain your balance.

Try doing yoga for stress relief by doing parts of a full routine. If you are pressed for time, these techniques will fit into your life well.

Deep Breathing - If you want to instantly unwind and revive, do deep breathing. Most people most of the time breathe through the chest. This shallow breathing is caused by tension and stress.

Breathing deeply through the belly oxygenates the muscles thereby relieving tension. Fill up your lower abdomen by breathing in. Contract the same area by breathing out. Do the breathing through your nose. This is the easiest part of doing yoga for stress relief.

Meditation - Spend a few minutes a day quieting your mind. It sounds difficult with a hectic schedule. Take a few minutes to sit in a quiet place. You can close your office door at work or go in your bathroom at home and lock the door. Sit comfortably and close your eyes.

Breathe deeply and focus on the area between and just above the bridge of your nose. This is the third eye (eye of the soul). When a thought comes to your mind, envision it with wings and let it fly away. Do this until you are relaxed and centered.

CHAPTER 10

Yoga Poses For Stress Relief

Feelings of being overwhelmed can leave you feeling stretched, undervalued and struggling to meet all the demands placed on you. When you feel like this, what do you?

Do you come home and slump on the sofa and snack on fast food? Or go for a drink with your colleagues and end up spending money you do not have and panic how you are going to make it through the next few days?

If you are a yoga beginner, you have probably heard that it is good to practice yoga as a way to cope with stress and stressful situations.

There are numerous health benefits from practicing yoga as a form of stress relief, these include reduced feelings of anxiety and worry, slower respiratory and heart rates and it can also help soothe tension related headaches and eyestrain.

The following simple yoga sequence is ideal for you to practice in the evenings to help you unwind from the stresses of your day. As with all exercises, please consult your doctor if you have any medical conditions and show respect and patience with your body.

1. The Child Pose. A classic yoga pose which gently stretches the whole spine and calms and soothes your mind. Kneel on the floor with your knees together and sit back on your heels. Stretch your trunk forward over your thighs and rest your forehead on the floor.

Place your arms back beside your body with your palms facing up so your hands are resting by your feet.

If this feels uncomfortable, spread your knees apart and rest a small cushion between your thighs and then sit on your heels and stretch your trunk forward as before. Breathe slowly and deeply for at least 2 - 3 minutes.

2. Downward Facing Dog Pose. A beautiful pose which rejuvenates the whole spine. Bringing your head low increases the blood flow to your brain and helps to clear and calm your mind.

Start on your hands and knees with your knees directly under your hips and your hands in line with your shoulders, fingers facing forward. Lift your hips and stretch the legs, heels down. Press the palms of your hands down. Relax and open and broaden your shoulders. Stay in this pose for 5 - 10 breaths.

3. Mountain Pose / Tadasana. The mountain pose helps to ground your energy and teaches you correct posture, balance and encourages you to be still, steady and strong - even when your mind is all over the place.

The mountain pose helps to calm and steady your nerves. Stand with your feet together. If it is comfortable for you, have the big toes, inner ankles and inner heels touching.

Spread the weight evenly over the feet. Tighten your kneecaps and pull up the thigh muscles and your lower abdomen. Breathe and feel your spine lengthening, let your tailbone sink and lift in front of the body. Feel your chest opening.

Allow your arms to hang down the sides of the body with the palms facing the legs, fingers gently extending towards the floor. Relax your shoulders and allow your shoulder blades to slide down. Relax your face, lengthen the back of your neck and look straight ahead. Stay steady in this pose for 3 - 10 rounds of deep abdominal breathing.

4. Corpse Pose. Lie on the floor on your back, arms stretched out a

few inches from the sides of your body with the palms facing up. Have your feet slightly wider apart than your hips and relax your ankles.

Gently close your eyes and allow your whole body to relax. Stay still for at least 5 - 10 minutes. Slowly stretch your body, roll over to your side and come up to a comfortable sitting position.

This simple yoga sequence is ideal for yoga beginners to help you to relax, release tension and relieve stress, especially at the end of a busy day. Enjoy.

5 CHAIR POSE

Take a seat, sit up straight, relax your shoulders, chest, and let your stomach relax, as if you're just letting all flop to your feet.

Take a deep and slow breath in from your diaphragm, feel the oxygen move up through your body, and then exhale slowly for the same time you done when you inhaled.

That's the breathing element of chair yoga.

6. Butterfly Pose - Sit on the floor with your knees out and soles of the feet touching - like a butterfly. Keeping your back straight and holding your feet, slowly raise and lower your knees several times. Then, lean forward from your hips. Hold this pose for a few minutes while breathing normally.

CHAPTER 11

Yoga For Beginners To Ease Knee Pain

The knee is wonderful simple machine, a coming together of bone, ligaments, cartilage, and muscle that can either make physical activity a joy or turn it into pure misery. The knee is also extremely sensitive to pressure when someone new is beginning a yoga routine. It's important to make sure you are in a yoga for beginners class.

The knee is made up of three bones: the end of the femur (the thighbone), the patella (or kneecap) and the end of the tibia (or shinbone). Between the tibia and the femur are two pads of cartilage that cushion the area and act as shock absorbers.

The bones and cartilage are all held together and aligned by two sets of ligaments called the cruciates and the collaterals that crisscross behind the kneecap and run alongside of the knee. The large muscles of the leg help to support the ligaments and keep everything in place.

One thing that leads to knee injuries is the fact that today's activities and exercises are a bit beyond the scope of what the knee is designed to handle. Therefore, it is important to keep in mind that in injury recovery as well as injury and disease prevention, the muscles that support the knee should be balanced.

Yoga is particularly beneficial in doing this because it engages the leg muscles evenly and requires a focus on balance. This is particularly important in regards to yoga for beginners. Yoga also contributes to flexibility, which is not only important for the muscles, but is also important to keep your cartilage spongy and cushion-y.

As with all physical activity, there is a potential for injury, even with yoga, if you push too far and try to do more than what you're able to do. There are several things you can do to protect yourself against damage to your knees.

1- First, you should avoid hyperextending your knees. This is sometimes easy to do in certain standing poses like the [Triangle Pose] and the [Extended Leg Forward Bend], as well as seated forward bend stretches. Try to keep a slight bend in the knee as you are executing these poses.

2- Also, don't be afraid to use props. Rolled up towels and yoga blocks can come in handy to prevent you from asking more of your knees than they are able to give. If you are in a yoga for beginners class, props should be mandatory.

3- Focus on balance and engaging the muscles equally. Many knee injuries are caused by an imbalance in muscle development that throws the ligaments and knee bones out of alignment. Regular yoga practice helps prevent this by working and strengthening all muscles equally.

4- Focus on proper technique. Remember that improper body alignment is the reason for many strains and injuries. Keeping your body and your knees properly aligned is key to getting the most benefits out of your yoga practice.

5- Finally, listen to your body. Know when to push yourself, but also know when to pull back. Be aware that your knees don't always tell you immediately when you've overdone it.

A little discomfort is expected, but you should never continue if you're experiencing pain. If it hurts, it's time to stop or pull back. If you are in a yoga for beginners class, make sure your instructor is trained and aware of your newness to yoga.

Listen to your body. Know when to push yourself, but also know when to pull back. Be aware that your knees don't always tell you immediately when you've overdone it.

If you are in the yoga for beginners category, take your time to develop your practice. This slow approach will accustom your knees to the added pressure of such poses as chair and warrior II.

CHAPTER 12

How To Turn Yoga Into A Habit

A relaxing activity to enjoy is yoga- "A Hindu discipline aimed at training the consciousness for a state of perfect spiritual insight and tranquility". As long as you can stick to your goal of doing yoga everyday, you will feel more relaxed and will start to enjoy life one day at a time.

1. Set aside a time and place for yoga. Write it down in a notebook and set a reminder on your phone, just remember to get up and do your Yoga at that time.

Sooner or later it will go from a habit, to a lifestyle, and then transform to who you are. Find a place that is quiet and where you can focus on your inner strength and inner self. Yoga is about relaxing and unwinding, and you will not be able to do that with a bunch of kids running around.

2. Get well prepared for your yoga session. Put on comfortable, loose clothes (such as parachute pants and a workout tee.) Yoga is about free movement, so you need clothes that will allow for you to thoroughly enjoy the poses.

As well, it is best to practice yoga on an empty stomach, so it is advised to practice before breakfast. If you feel the need to eat, drink warm milk with honey to ease your stomach.

3. Find your starting position. I generally start with my feet crossed and my hands rested on my knees. I do so by grabbing my left foot and bringing it high onto my right thigh, then taking my right foot and resting it on my left thigh. Take deep breathes and

focus on your breathing for one minute.

4. Mountain Pose. Gradually stand up, feet together, shoulders relaxed, and weight evenly distributed through your soles. Place your arms at your side. Take a deep breath and raise your hands over your head, palms facing each other. With arms straight, stand tall and reach for the sky. Hold for 30 seconds and gradually lower arms.

5. Downward Dog. Start on all fours. Walk your hands forward and spread finger wide. Curl your toes under, and slowly press hips toward ceiling. Your body will look like an inverted V. Feet should be hip-width apart, and knees slightly bent. Hold this pose for 3 breaths.

6. Warrior. Stand with legs 3 to 4 feet apart, with your right foot turned out 90 degrees and your left foot tilted in slightly.

Starting with your hands at your hips, relax your shoulders, and extend them horizontally with palms down. Bend your right knee 90 degrees (keeping it over ankle) and gaze over the right hand. While practicing on your breathing, hold for one minute. Switch sides and repeat.

7. Tree Pose. Starting with arms at sides, shift your weight to your left leg and place the sole of your right foot inside left thigh. Once you are balanced, bring hands in front of you and do a prayer position (palms together.) Release your breath, and extend arms over shoulder, palms separated and facing each other. Hold for thirty seconds, lower and repeat on opposite side.

8. Bridge Pose Lie on back on floor with knees bend and directly over heels. With palms down, place hands at side, exhale, then press feet into floor as you lift your hips. Clasp your hands under lower back and press arms down, lifting your hips until thighs are parallel to floor, chest being brought towards chin. Hold for 1 minute. Don't forget to focus on breathing.

9. Triangle Pose. Standing with feet 3 feet apart and toes on your right foot turned 90 degree (left foot at 45 degrees,) extend arms

out to side and bend over your right leg.

Allow your right hand to touch the floor, or if it's more comfortable, rest it right below or above the knee. Extend your left hand fingertips above head, and reach for the ceiling. Turn head towards ceiling and hold for 5 breaths. Repeat on other side.

10. Seated Twist. Sit on the floor with legs extended. Cross right foot over outside of left thigh and bend the left knee. Keep the right knee pointed toward ceiling. Place left elbow to the outside of the right knee and right hand on the floor behind you.

Twist to the right, as far as you can. Keep both sides of your butt on the floor and try to move from your abdomen. Breathe and stay for 1 minute. Switch sides and repeat.

11. Cobra. Lie face down on the floor, thumbs directly under shoulders. Extend your legs with the tops of your feet on the floor. Tuck hips downward and squeeze your glutes. Press shoulders down and away from ears, while raising chest toward the wall in front of you. Relax and repeat five times.

12. Pigeon Pose. Start in a push-up position, palms under shoulders. Place your left knee on the floor near your shoulders with left heel by right hip. Lower down to your forearms and bring right leg down with the top of the foot on the floor.

While keeping chest lifted, gaze down. Pull belly button in toward spine and tighten pelvic-floor muscles; contract right side of glutes. Bend knee to floor and release. Do 5 reps, and repeat. Keep focusing on breathing.

13. Child's Pose (Another Favorite) Sit up comfortably on your heels. Roll your torso forward, bringing your forehead to rest on the floor in front of you. Lower your chest as close to your knee as possible (make sure you're comfortable) and extend arms in front of you. Hold this pose and breathe.

CHAPTER 13

Yoga For Improving Your Mind, Body And Spirit

Yoga for beginners is for everyone all ages, shapes and sizes. You first start out in Yoga as a novice and progress upwards until you are a master in the art.

In my opinion I call it an art as Yoga for beginners is about a combination of exercise combined with meditation and therefore it is much more than just running on a treadmill or lifting some weights. In fact the exercises associated with

Yoga are not in the modern sense traditional, you don't need to go down the gym but I would advise those of you newbies to go to a qualified instructor to start with. Exercises involve postures and balance plus controlled breathing as opposed to strength and speed or aerobic type training in other disciplines.

It is important for me to point out the fact that there are many different types of Yoga out there. They all have the same aim in mind and that is to improve mind, body and spirit. Some emphasize more or less on different on the main areas such as meditation, nutrition or exercise.

The most common form in the Western world is Hatha Yoga. This has come about due to the fact it is the most applicable to our western culture and westerners associate more readily with the methods involved.

I would suggest before beginning Yoga you briefly investigate the different varieties and pick the one that most matches in with your lifestyle.

If you don't have a local class you can go to then Yoga for beginners can be learned through instructional DVDs, books and multimedia as well as online. So it is easy to start.

You don't really need any equipment. Although a good yoga mat or yoga blanket is recommended. When you are ready to begin find a quiet spot in your house and follow the exercise plan you have decided upon. Can't be easier than that.

Some people prefer relaxing music when practicing their yoga meditation and exercises. Normally yoga is done without shoes or socks on but there are special socks you can buy that don't slip if you prefer. All forms of Yoga give benefits to health.

They combine the elements of exercise through postures, controlled breathing exercises and meditation as previously mentioned but you need to be clear what Yoga is ultimately about. Regular practice is great for strengthening mind and body.

Beginners of Yoga, will find almost immediate benefit when starting and this can very often be seen within the first two weeks or even less. Most people are surprised by the quick results they achieve within such a short time.

Yoga for beginners is like everything else that involves movement of the body. You should always start with a gentle warm up. Stretching gently is also important. Find a place where you won't be disturbed.

The length of time required varies and can depend greatly upon the level you are on. I personally use on average around 1/2 hour a day. When you do it is up to you. For me the best time is first thing in the morning but this is not always possible in the week so after work is my usual time.

To get the most out of Yoga it should become part of your lifestyle. Many beginners in Yoga find it helps them to unwind and relax. They find it invigorating and calming. It also improves their body's suppleness and muscular tonality.

CHAPTER 14

Basic Yoga Routines For Beginners

Finding time for relaxation can be difficult. We can look forward to the weekends but sometimes even those are so busy we still can't relax. Long working hours added together with other preoccupations leave little time to relax and reflect. Yet these things are important to our health.

Yoga is a practice that refreshes both the mind and body and just a few moments devoted to it every day can bring about a marked change in one's life. Yoga for weight loss is also becoming quite popular. However there are a number of things you should know before you begin your yoga exercise. These tips can actually be quite helpful for beginners.

• Be Peaceful: The primary objective is to give peace to the mind and the body. Hence it is important to keep out unwanted thoughts that jumble up our minds. Try to clear your mind before committing to any yoga exercise. This will improve your concentration and enable you to practice yoga in a better way.

• Be Silly: It is important to feel free while practicing yoga. Being too self-conscious can stifle the learning curve as it stops us from making mistakes. No wonder they may be discomforting, mistakes actually make us learn. Ever wondered why children learn so quickly?

This is because they make a lot of mistakes. Moreover, realize that when you are beginning, you are bound to fall many times. Even if you are getting better, you will still fall. Fretting about this and feeling embarrassed only takes the joy out of yoga and makes us too shy to practice it in its full capacity.

• Be Consistent: Whatever routine we set for ourselves, it is important that we stick to it on a consistent basis. Even if we give it just 5 minutes of our time every day, we must be sure not to miss a routine.

Inconsistency drastically slows down learning and is also a sign that we are not committed to the exercise. However try not to get too disciplined about yoga as it is more about loving ourselves then being all rigid and regimented. Moreover, the emphasis should be on working smart, rather than working hard.

• Be Real: Finally, realize that yoga is about staying in touch with reality, rather than floating on a cloud. Sure it is a relaxing exercise, but that does not mean that we get lost in it. Be sure of your objective for practicing yoga so that you can stay focused.

CHAPTER 15

Considerations To Get The Most Out Of Your Yoga Practice

For myself and for many others, making time for yoga is the only time I take for myself to turn inward, get my sweat on, and oh does it replenish.

Some of the benefits of yoga are:

* Improved movement & flexibility

* Strength & posture improvements

* Circulation increase & lymphatic drainage

* Less stress

* Improved concentration

* Improved heart health

* and even relieves chronic medical conditions

While I have the deepest respect for the ancient practice, mind-body connection, and OM in spirit with my fellow yogis, I move and see through the eyes and body of a Strength and Conditioning Coach.

That being said, what I share with you in this chapter is to benefit your body first, and as a byproduct, your mind will soar into eternal bliss. That is my hope, anyway, and if you travel on a yogic path, you know or will soon know what I'm talking about.

Whether you want to begin a yoga practice or have been practicing for eternity, here are 4 considerations to get the most from your practice:

1. If it feels good...

If the stretch or pose feels amazing, chances are it's not the one you should focus on. Strength and flexibility improvements are never made by doing things that are easy. Take a few moments in your favorite position to grab the bliss, but spend more time on the ones that stump you and challenge you.

2. Take the road less traveled...

This is very important. Taking the road less traveled means to go the other direction. How do you spend most of your day?

If you are in a seated, slumped over position such as at a computer, your road less traveled is one that takes you to a standing, back bending, heart opening place. Conversely, people who stand up all day will want to journey into forward folding and lengthening the muscles in the back of their body.

3. Ask and ye shall receive...

So how does a yoga instructor know what road the students have been traveling all day? They don't. Speak up and request certain stretches, poses, or directions. A quality yoga instructor will adapt to the students and believe me, they love the interaction.

Requests invite conversation, create a community environment, and many bodies will benefit. Chances are some of your fellow yogis have been traveling down that same road all day.

4. Try as you will...

There are numerous poses, progressions, and regressions in yoga so you will be challenged. Personally, yoga will be a practice I don't expect to perfect...ever. However, if you are looking for benefits such as an increase in lean muscle mass or fat loss, you will have to do some cross training and tweak your nutrition habits.

It is true that many yoga practitioners look great. This is because of many reasons including yoga. Yoga and other body-weight-only training, will only improve muscle endurance. To gain lean muscle mass thus provide the opportunity to burn more body fat, you must add progressive resistance and you must burn more fuel than consumed.

CHAPTER 16

Choosing Yoga Equipment As A Beginner

Yoga is about being relaxed and calm, and if you want to perform at your best, you will need to have the right equipment. You'll need to learn about the various types of equipment as well as determining where you can get your yoga equipment. If you want to purchase your equipment online, there are some great websites for all of your yoga needs.

Mats are typically the first item that anyone buys when starting out with yoga. You'll need a high-quality mat that is sturdy and doesn't move around while you are involved in yoga.

It should be thick as well as comfortable to sit on. The mat should be long enough so that when you are lying down to do a yoga pose; your head or legs are not hanging off the mat.

Yoga blocks are normally made of foam material, but they can be made from wood as well. These are used to relieve some of the pressure from poses where you are standing up. They are also useful for poses where you put your hands or head on the floor.

Yoga blankets are used in several different ways. During meditation, they are used to place over your head to make the mediation process seem more surreal.

Blankets are also used for stability while you are in a sitting pose. Use a yoga blanket that is colorful and pleasing to your eye. You want the blanket to be made of materials that are not itchy or uncomfortable.

Meditation cushions will keep you comfortable in a sitting position while you meditate. There are several kinds of meditation cushions, and you should purchase one that fits your body type, is comfortable for you to sit on, and is well-made.

Yoga Relaxation Eyebags

Yoga eyebags can be made infused with lavender to promote a deeper relaxation. You simply place them over your eyes to block out light when you are laying down in relaxation pose.

Strap

Straps are very useful to help you "stretch that extra bit more" in a challenging pose, for example in the seated forward bend you can place a strap around the soles of your feet and hold the strap as you stretch forward.

Sandbag

This is an interesting prop to use. You place a sandbag on parts of the body, this helps to deepen your posture.

A Chair

Absolutely essential for students who are very inflexible, maybe overweight, disabled or elderly people who are exercising for the first time. Seated yoga enables you to do the same pose as the rest of your class, participate at your own level and still be part of a regular class example, you can do seated cobra whilst the rest of the class does the full floor yoga pose.

If you feel too old, stiff or disabled in some way, try to use a yoga prop. it will give you the extra support and assistance you may need to deepen your yoga practice.

CHAPTER 17

Yoga For Overall Health And Weight Management

Today more and more people are recognizing the importance of yoga for health. As a result more and more people are incorporating yoga into their workout regime.

Yoga is a holistic approach to one's overall wellbeing. It is a scientific system of physical and mental exercises. Yoga originated in India some 3000 years ago.

Over the years it has been defined and refined by various yoga gurus. Overall, it consists of various asanas (poses) and Pranayama (breathing exercises). Regular practice of asanas and breathing exercises results in overall improvement in one's health.

Yoga poses and breathing exercises are designed to provide stimulation to each and every parts of the human body. Yoga poses not only make the body strong, supple, flexible, balanced and healthy, but they also help improve mental concentration.

According to ancient yogis, improvement in mental concentration helps bring about overall improvement in one's health. Yoga helps bring about mental peace, which in turn helps reduce stress. Today stress is one of the main contributors of many lifestyle diseases like, heart problems, high blood pressure, etc.

Yoga For Weight Management

Thus yoga for health is not just a statement, it is a fact. However, yoga does not just help bring about overall improvement in the functioning of our organs and body parts; it also plays a very important role in weight management.

Obesity is a very common problem in America. Many of the lifestyle diseases, like high blood pressure, high cholesterol, heart diseases, diabetes, etc are linked to obesity. Yoga for health combined with an active lifestyle greatly helps in burning excess fat.

So how exactly does it help reduce weight? Yoga helps to improve our metabolism. Metabolism refers to the chemical processes in our body that help to transform food into energy. Metabolism is regulated by the thyroid gland. Various yoga poses, especially those that involve the neck area, help to improve our metabolism.

Poses such as the camel pose, rabbit pose, shoulder stand and bridge pose are specifically designed to help improve the functioning of our thyroid gland. When our metabolism improves, it helps to burn more calories.

And when you combine this with healthy eating habits, you experience an overall reduction in your weight. Moreover, an improvement in your metabolism also results in you feeling more energetic.

According to yoga for health experts, when you combine a balanced and healthy diet with yoga, you get a holistic weight loss program. A balanced diet should consist of fiber rich food, vegetables, fruits, whole grains, and protein. One should restrict the intake of processed food and high fat food if one is serious about losing weight.

Regular practice of yoga not only helps one maintain proper weight, but also provides numerous health benefits. It assists improved blood circulation, better concentration, improves stamina, flexibility and body strength. Regular practice of yoga helps to treat many illnesses like, high blood pressure, diabetes, high cholesterol, arthritis, joint problems, etc.

Today most people lead a stressful life. In today's competitive environment we have to constantly exert ourselves to prove that we are good. The pressure of work and life causes a lot of stress. By taking up yoga for health one can achieve better health and mental peace.

CHAPTER 18

Must Know Information For You As A Beginner

Yoga for beginners may be a bit challenging at first, but once you've gotten used to the different yoga poses and techniques, it will be a fun, continuous learning process. If you've decided to practice yoga, here are important things you should understand before you start:

1. It is vital that you consult with your health care provide first

Even if you only plan on practicing less aggressive styles of yoga, it is still recommended that you check with your doctor first if you have any underlying chronic conditions as well as bone or muscle injuries.

Yoga for beginners is still a new physical fitness program that needs your doctor's approval no matter how relaxing you think it may be. Remember, safety should always be your top priority to avoid injury.

2. Yoga is for everyone

Contrary to popular belief, yoga isn't just for fit and flexible individuals. In fact, anyone can practice the art - young or old, slim or heavy and even flexible or not. As mentioned above, yoga is a continuous learning process.

You don't have to feel discouraged every time you can't perform a pose right. The practice is all about exploring your inner self through different styles of yoga so don't hold back and just keep on practicing.

3. Start slow

With all the wonderful things you might have heard or read about the practice, it's easy to get excited and dive right in. Doing so may just burn out your body faster or result to injuries so it's important to take things slow and follow your natural learning pace.

Learn and master all the basics first before trying out more complicated poses or techniques. More importantly, if you're attending a yoga for beginners class, let your instructor guide you through the learning process - follow his instructions and don't try to get ahead.

4. Keeping a journal to track your progress is important

Keeping a record of everything you learn about yoga will do nothing but good to your progress. After a month or so, reading your journal will show you how much you've improved as a yogi. Yoga also has LOTS of terminologies so it doesn't hurt to write them down.

5. Yoga is a lifestyle, not a "diet" that ends

Many people treat yoga like a weight loss diet, stopping once the desired weight is achieved then resuming when the weight is gained back. Yoga shouldn't be approached as all or nothing. When you decide to practice yoga, it is important to understand that it is more than a physical fitness program - it is a lifestyle that will improve your general well-being.

6. What Style to Choose?

There are many different styles of yoga to choose from. Gyms and studios usually offer hatha and vinyasa yoga for beginners classes. The word hatha actually refers to yoga in general, as all yoga styles are hatha yoga. However, classes referred to as hatha are usually slower paced, gentle, and focused on the basics of stretching and breathing in different poses.

Vinyasa classes involve more movement and are more vigorous. Both of these are okay for beginners. Just remember to find classes labeled as yoga for beginners.

There are many styles of yoga to choose from and choosing the right style for you will have an impact on whether you stick with it or not. Try different styles and teachers until you find one that resonates with you.

Look into the different styles, which include hatha, vinyasa, ashtanga, power, iyengar, kundalini, bikram, hot yoga, anusara, jivamukti, forrest, kripalu, integral, moksha, sivananda, laughter, and others.

7. Where to Start... Home, Gym, or Studio?

Learning from an actual, live teacher can't be beat, so taking a yoga for beginners class at a local gym or studio is best. Classes at gyms typically focus more on the physical workout that yoga provides while classes at yoga studios involve more mind, body, spirit aspects like meditation, breathing, and chanting in addition to asanas.

If you don't have the resources or desire to start with a class, the best thing to do is get a yoga for beginners DVD for use at home.

Yoga books and yoga card decks work well for learning more about technique and specifics of poses, but starting with a yoga for beginners DVD will be easier as it requires less effort on your part. There are also many great yoga for beginners resources online like virtual classes and step by step guides.

8. What Do You Need?

You will need a yoga mat and comfortable clothes that fit properly and are not too big. That's it. That is all you really need. In addition, you might want to have a couple of blocks, a strap, and a towel or yoga rug depending on what type of class or style you choose, but a yoga mat and comfortable clothes are all you really need to begin.

9. Things To Do and Know When Taking Classes:

Shoes off: You should take off your shoes when entering a yoga studio. This helps keep the space clean. Yoga is done barefoot, without shoes or socks.

Cell phones off: Before entering the facility, power your cell phone off.

Arrive on time: Arrive at least ten minutes prior to class so that you have time to check in, put your things away, talk to the teacher, and set out your mat.

Let the instructor know you are a beginner/new: Talk to the instructor so s/he knows that you are new or a beginner and if you would like help.

Stay for the whole class: Refrain from leaving in the middle of class as it is rude to the teacher and disruptive to the class. If you decide you don't like the class or the teacher it is proper etiquette to stay until the end.

Don't skip savasana: This is the final resting pose and is one of the most important and most enjoyable. A lot of people discover that it is one of their favorite poses.

Put the above tips and tools to work for you and you'll be comfortable with your yoga practice in no time. For more information on yoga for beginners.

CHAPTER 19

Tips For Yoga Classes

Regardless of which specific version of Yoga you choose to practice, there are a number of things that apply to Yoga universally, rather than to individual branches of the discipline.

If you want to get the most from your Yoga classes, you will begin to learn to understand these things and develop them into your own Yoga routine. There are a number of different reasons for taking up Yoga.

Broadly, people are looking for one of three things: physical health, mental health or spiritual health. All three are important and all three are realistic goals in a Yoga class.

Whatever it is you are trying to achieve through Yoga there will be always be a class and style that will be suitable for you. You can research in a library, online or even by asking various Yoga instructors, and this will help you find the type of Yoga that will match the best results for you individually.

You also want to check and make sure that the instructor knows what they are doing and what they are teaching. You don't want to be pushed too fast or beyond your capabilities and most important you do not want to suffer any injuries.

Choose your class wisely and make sure that there are no hidden costs involved. Pay as you go may be the best choice for you. You'll want to know what to expect and you'll want to take it slowly at first when you do begin.

Yoga is also great for your circulation and for weight loss. Your diet is especially important as well for your health. Your approach to fitness and well-being and to life in general should be nonviolent one - working smoothly with concentration and determination at your own pace without competing with anyone else. This isn't a competition.

Take your time and do it correctly. Remember, this is a marathon, not a sprint. Breathing is so important in yoga. Just as one stressful situation goes into your next challenge, relaxing for a few minutes every day gradually carries over into the rest of your daily life and activities.

Each day you will feel more relaxed. Yoga is wonderful for all ages and does great things for one's body and mind. If you need to relieve stress as well, then give yoga a try.

If you are a Yoga teacher or an experienced practitioner, the following tips may be of use to your students or friends. By now, almost everyone has probably heard about the benefits of Yoga.

Everyone probably knows someone, a friend of a friend, or a relative, who practices Yoga and raves about it. Perhaps they have even thought about trying it themselves, but dismissed it.

Yoga can often feel intimidating to beginners, mostly because of all the unknown factors. Truth be told, beginners have nothing to fear. Yoga for beginners is a non-intimidating, welcoming environment where interested people can learn the techniques and lifestyle, which we know improves the quality of life.

Check with a Doctor

As it is with any other form of movement, people should always check with their doctors before beginning to practice Yoga. Perhaps there are specific health concerns the Yoga teacher should be aware of, or poses to be avoided because of an injury or tender area.

Pregnant women should always let the instructor know of their condition as well, because some of the poses must be adapted to accommodate the growing fetus. However, to be safe, pregnant students should practice with a certified prenatal Yoga instructor in a specialized class.

Equipment and Clothing

Yoga requires very little in the way of clothing and equipment. Many Yoga centers provide mats, blocks, and straps for participants to use. Some people prefer to use their own mats, which can be purchased from a variety of sporting goods stores.

Blocks and straps are often helpful for students, who do not have the flexibility to perform some of the postures. Again, these are often provided by the Yoga facility, but can certainly be purchased.

Yoga students should wear comfortable clothing that moves with the body. Loose t-shirts and pants can pose problems during certain poses, as they ride down the belly or up the leg.

Most Yoga-inspired clothing is a blend of cotton and spandex, to provide soft, comfortable clothing that hugs the body. Most importantly, participants should wear what they are comfortable in, and clothing that poses little disruption to the postures.

Beginner Yoga classes move slowly, ensuring that all participants learn how to perform each technique properly. Yoga teachers often demonstrate the technique, talking about how it should feel, and other important cues to watch for.

Then, the students practice it with the teacher or the teacher walks around the room to make sure each student is practicing correctly. The connection between the teacher and the student should be constant. In other words: A teacher should observe and communicate with students at all times.

Yoga instructors are trained to watch the students carefully, to determine who needs extra support, or to help if there is a problem with safety or alignment.

Students will find that the soothing environment and the careful guidance of the Yoga teacher creates a positive experience during classes. People of all physical abilities can attend a beginner's Yoga class and succeed with gentle guidance.

CONCLUSION

Yoga is an excellent way to stay healthy and fit. It is not only good for your physical health but for emotional, mental and spiritual health as well. Learning yoga is indeed a step by step process.

It is always better to start with some easy asanas or postures so that you get motivation to continue. The simplest yoga asanas are similar to the day to day activities like lying down, standing or sitting in different positions but in an orderly fashion which proves to be beneficial for health.

Even doctors and medical practitioners recommend practicing yoga regularly because of its great therapeutic benefits. If you are a beginner, then you will be pleased to see great results instantly.

Some of the most recommended yoga for beginners include vini-yoga or kripalu yoga. One you have a strong command on these simple yoga asanas, you can move onto advanced yoga asanas like Ashtanga yoga or power yoga.

You can practice for around 10-15 minutes at an initial stage which will help in increasing the flexibility of the muscle joints, enhance lubrication and improve blood circulation in the body. This will prepare your body for more complex yoga asana. It is very important to have a correct and erect body posture while practicing yoga.

Breathing exercises are a significant aspect of yoga for beginners. Some of the most effective breathing exercises include Anuloma-viloma, pranayama and kapalbharti. These exercises help in improving the breathing pattern and increases lung capacity.

These exercises will make you feel relaxed and rejuvenated. They are great stress busters and provides you relief from day to day tensions, worries and anxieties.

If you are a beginner then it is very important for you to have basic knowledge of yoga etiquettes. The yoga teachers play a very important role in teaching some simple yoga asanas and basic etiquettes of yoga.

A beginner should always start with simple and basic yoga stretches like finishing postures, back bends, balance postures, supine, twist, sitting or standing positions.

It is very important for you to let your yoga teacher know that you are a beginner so that he/she pays special attention to you until you get a hold on various yoga asanas. Before practicing yoga, it is always better to take a nice bath and it is advisable to end your yoga session with shavasana.

Avoid having food before 3-4 hours of your yoga class. Don't overeat. Wear loose and comfortable clothes for yoga classes so that your body feels free. Have some water before the class starts.

As a beginner, all you need to get set for yoga for beginners are a yoga mat and comfortable loose clothes. You can join any reputable yoga classes near to your home so that you can commute easily. There are different types of yoga asana.

It is very important for you to get basic knowledge of all the yoga stretches and then get a control over them one by one.

Yoga is a gentle, peaceful but very effective exercise. It is an excellent option for regular practice. Yoga stretches, purifies and heals the body. Practicing Yoga regularly keeps the body supple and prevents its deterioration. Various poses of Yoga strengthen and tone the muscles. Besides increasing the flexibility of joints and muscles, it also massages internal organs and glands.

Yoga for beginners is a simple system of stretching exercises. As you progress learning Yoga from a professional trainer, you realize how Yoga helps to develop inner physical strength and stamina. These simple exercises aid holistic wellness.

As a beginner, you must choose simpler forms of Yoga poses and should slowly graduate to more complex ones. When you begin Yoga exercises should be of shorter duration and with lesser body stress. Slowly these beginners' exercises can be replaced with more complex exercises and longer duration.

Yoga is therapeutic by nature. Traditional yoga practiced in the right environment and under proper supervision, creates harmony between mind and body and leads to healing. Through yoga practice, all of the layers become cleansed and balanced.

Made in the USA
Middletown, DE
30 May 2019